Push Past 50

50

Building Muscle with Bodyweight Exercises

By

Alex Lenero

Contents

Introduction

As men approach their 50s, they may start to feel like they are past their prime and that building muscle is an unattainable goal. However, this couldn't be further from the truth. With the right approach and mindset, building muscle at 50 is possible and can bring numerous physical and mental benefits.

In this book, "Push Past 50: Building Muscle with Bodyweight Exercises," we will explore the principles of bodyweight training and show you how to use push-up exercises and other bodyweight workouts to build muscle, increase strength, and improve overall fitness. You will learn how to set realistic goals, understand the science behind bodyweight training, and stay motivated throughout your fitness journey.

This book is designed for men and women over 50 who want to take control of their health and fitness. Whether you are a seasoned fitness enthusiast or just starting out, this book provides a comprehensive guide to building muscle and improving your overall fitness with bodyweight exercises. So, let's get started!

The Benefits of Bodyweight Training for Men Over 50

The Benefits of Bodyweight Training for Men Over 50:

1. Convenience: Bodyweight exercises can be done anywhere, at any time, and do not require any equipment or gym membership. This makes it easy for men over 50 to incorporate bodyweight workouts into their daily routines.

2. Increased Strength: Bodyweight exercises, such as push-ups, squats, and lunges, target multiple muscle groups, helping to increase overall strength and muscle mass.

3. Improved Balance and Coordination: Bodyweight exercises, such as single-leg squats and balance work, help to improve balance and coordination, reducing the risk of falls and injury.

4. Better Flexibility and Mobility: Bodyweight exercises, such as stretching and yoga, can help to improve flexibility and mobility, reducing the risk of injury and making daily activities easier.

5. Cost-Effective: Bodyweight exercises do not require any equipment or gym membership, making it an affordable and cost-effective way to get in shape and build muscle.

6. Mental Health: Exercise, including bodyweight training, has been shown to have a positive impact

on mental health, reducing stress and anxiety and improving overall well-being.

Setting Realistic Goals

One of the keys to success in bodyweight training is setting realistic goals. When setting your goals, it's important to consider your current fitness level, your health history, and any limitations you may have. Here are some tips for setting realistic goals:

1. Start Slow: If you're just starting out, it's important to start slow and gradually build up your strength and endurance. Don't try to do too much too soon, as this can lead to injury and burnout.

2. Be Specific: Instead of setting vague goals like "I want to get in shape," set specific, measurable goals such as "I want to be able to do 10 push-ups in a row."

3. Set Reasonable Time Frames: Give yourself enough time to achieve your goals, but don't set unrealistic time frames that are unlikely to be met.

4. Celebrate Small Wins: Celebrate each small win along the way, as this will help keep you motivated and on track.

5. Revisit and Adjust: Regularly revisit your goals and adjust them as needed. As you get stronger and more confident, you may want to set new, more challenging goals.

By setting realistic goals and celebrating small wins, you'll be more likely to stay motivated and on track, making it easier to achieve your long-term fitness goals.

Understanding the Science of Bodyweight Training

The science of bodyweight training is based on the principles of progressive resistance training, which involves gradually increasing the difficulty of your exercises over time. This allows your muscles to adapt and grow stronger, leading to improved overall fitness and muscle mass.

Here are some key concepts to understand when it comes to the science of bodyweight training:

1. Progressive Resistance Training: This involves gradually increasing the difficulty of your exercises over time, allowing your muscles to adapt and grow stronger.

2. Muscle Adaptation: Your muscles adapt to the stress placed on them during exercise, leading to increased strength and muscle mass.

3. Time Under Tension: The amount of time your muscles are under tension during an exercise is important in building muscle. Bodyweight exercises, such as push-ups, allow you to control the amount of time your muscles are under tension, making them an effective way to build muscle.

4. Variety is Key: To get the most out of bodyweight training, it's important to vary your exercises and target different muscle groups. This helps to

prevent boredom and ensures that all muscle groups are being worked equally.

By understanding the science behind bodyweight training, you'll be better equipped to design effective workout routines and achieve your fitness goals.

The Principles of Progressive Resistance Training

Progressive resistance training is a key principle in bodyweight training, and involves gradually increasing the difficulty of your exercises over time. This allows your muscles to adapt and grow stronger, leading to improved overall fitness and muscle mass. Here are the key principles of progressive resistance training:

1. Gradual Increase in Difficulty: The difficulty of your exercises should be gradually increased over time, allowing your muscles to adapt and grow stronger. This can be done by increasing the number of repetitions, sets, or by adding weight to your exercises.

2. Consistency: Consistency is key when it comes to progressive resistance training. Regular exercise, even if it is at a low intensity, is better than sporadic, high-intensity workouts.

3. Overloading: Overloading your muscles is an important aspect of progressive resistance training. This involves gradually increasing the weight or difficulty of your exercises, putting more stress on your muscles, and forcing them to adapt and grow stronger.

4. Rest and Recovery: Rest and recovery are just as important as exercise when it comes to progressive resistance training. Adequate rest and recovery time allows your muscles to recover and

grow stronger, making it possible to increase the difficulty of your exercises over time.

How to Get the Most Out of Push-up Exercises

Push-up exercises are a staple of bodyweight training and can be a highly effective way to build muscle and improve overall fitness. Here are some tips for getting the most out of push-up exercises:

1. Proper Form: It's important to maintain proper form when doing push-ups to ensure that you are targeting the right muscle groups and reducing the risk of injury. Make sure to keep your body in a straight line, your core engaged, and your hands placed slightly wider than shoulder-width apart.

2. Vary Your Push-up Variations: To get the most out of push-up exercises, it's important to vary your push-up variations. This can be done by changing the hand placement, adding a stability ball, or using an unstable surface such as a BOSU ball.

3. Increase the Difficulty Over Time: To continue making progress, it's important to gradually increase the difficulty of your push-up exercises over time. This can be done by increasing the number of repetitions, sets, or by adding weight to your push-ups.

4. Focus on Quality Over Quantity: It's better to do a few push-ups with proper form than many push-ups with poor form. Focus on maintaining proper form and technique, even if it means doing fewer repetitions.

Push-ups are a classic exercise that is popular for good reason. Here are 10 benefits of push-ups:

1. Strengthens multiple muscle groups: Push-ups primarily work the chest, triceps, and shoulders, but they also engage the core, back, and leg muscles to help stabilize the body.

2. Builds upper body strength: Regular push-ups can increase upper body strength, helping you lift heavier objects and perform everyday tasks more easily.

3. Improves cardiovascular health: Push-ups are a great way to increase your heart rate, which can improve cardiovascular health.

4. Boosts metabolism: Push-ups can help increase your metabolism, which may help you burn more calories throughout the day.

5. Improves posture: Push-ups strengthen the muscles in the upper back and shoulders, which can improve posture and reduce the risk of back pain.

6. Enhances bone health: Regular strength training exercises like push-ups can help increase bone density, reducing the risk of osteoporosis.

7. Can be done anywhere: Push-ups are a versatile exercise that can be done virtually anywhere, requiring no equipment.

8. Improves balance and stability: Push-ups require you to maintain balance and stability, which can improve overall body control and coordination.

9. Increases endurance: Regular push-up training can increase muscular endurance, allowing you to perform more repetitions over time.

10. Mental benefits: Exercise like push-ups can boost mood, reduce stress, and improve overall mental health.

The Importance of Variety in Bodyweight Workouts

Variety is an important aspect of bodyweight training, and can help to prevent boredom, ensure that all muscle groups are being worked equally, and reduce the risk of injury. Here are some reasons why variety is important in bodyweight workouts:

1. Prevents Boredom: Doing the same exercises repeatedly can lead to boredom, making it less likely that you'll stick to your workout routine. By incorporating a variety of exercises into your routine, you'll be more likely to stay motivated and engaged.

2. Targets Different Muscle Groups: By varying your exercises, you'll be able to target different muscle groups, ensuring that all muscle groups are being worked equally. This helps to prevent muscle imbalances and reduces the risk of injury.

3. Increases Challenge: Varying your exercises can help to increase the challenge of your workouts, allowing you to continue making progress and reaching your fitness goals.

4. Improves Overall Fitness: Bodyweight workouts that incorporate a variety of exercises can help to improve overall fitness, including strength, endurance, flexibility, and balance.

Bodyweight Workouts for Men Over 50

Bodyweight workouts are an effective and convenient way for men over 50 to build muscle and improve overall fitness. Here are some types of bodyweight workouts that are particularly well-suited for men over 50:

1. Upper Body Workouts: Upper body workouts, such as push-ups and pull-ups, can help to build muscle and increase strength in the chest, arms, and back.

2. Core Workouts: Core workouts, such as planks and sit-ups, can help to build a strong, stable core, improving balance and reducing the risk of injury.

3. Lower Body Workouts: Lower body workouts, such as squats and lunges, can help to build muscle and increase strength in the legs and glutes.

4. Total Body Workouts: Total body workouts, such as burpees and jumping jacks, can help to build muscle and increase overall fitness, targeting multiple muscle groups at once.

5. Stretching and Yoga: Stretching and yoga can help to improve flexibility and mobility, reducing the risk of injury and making daily activities easier.

The Basics of Push-up Variations

Push-up exercises are a staple of bodyweight training, and there are numerous variations that can be used to target different muscle groups and increase the difficulty of the exercise. Here are some of the most common push-up variations:

1. Standard Push-ups: The standard push-up is a classic exercise that targets the chest, triceps, and core. To perform a standard push-up, start in a plank position with your hands placed slightly wider than shoulder-width apart and your body in a straight line. Lower your body until your chest touches the ground, then push back up to the starting position.

2. Diamond Push-ups: Diamond push-ups are a variation of the standard push-up that target the triceps. To perform a diamond push-up, place your hands together in a diamond shape and perform a push-up as you would with a standard push-up.

3. Wide-Arm Push-ups: Wide-arm push-ups are a variation of the standard push-up that target the chest. To perform a wide-arm push-up, place your hands wider than shoulder-width apart and perform a push-up as you would with a standard push-up.

4. Decline Push-ups: Decline push-ups are a variation of the standard push-up that target the chest and triceps. To perform a decline push-up, elevate your feet and perform a push-up as you would with a standard push-up.

5. Plyometric Push-ups: Plyometric push-ups are a
   dynamic variation of the standard push-up that
   target the chest, triceps, and core. To perform a
   plyometric push-up, push up explosively, lifting
   your hands off the ground, and clap before landing
   back in the starting position.

Upper Body Workouts

Upper body workouts are an effective way to build muscle and increase strength in the chest, arms, and back. Here are some bodyweight exercises that can be included in an upper body workout:

1. Push-ups: Push-ups are a classic exercise that target the chest, triceps, and core. There are numerous variations of push-ups, including standard, diamond, wide-arm, decline, and plyometric push-ups.

2. Pull-ups: Pull-ups are a challenging exercise that target the back, arms, and core. They can be performed using a pull-up bar or a resistance band.

3. Dips: Dips are an exercise that target the triceps and shoulders. They can be performed using parallel bars or a sturdy chair.

4. Chin-ups: Chin-ups are a variation of pull-ups that target the back, arms, and biceps. They can be performed using a pull-up bar or a resistance band.

5. Plank to Push-up: The plank to push-up is a dynamic exercise that targets the chest, triceps, and core. To perform a plank to push-up, start in a plank position, then push up into a push-up position, and then return to the plank position.

Core Workouts

Core workouts are an effective way to build a strong, stable core, improving balance and reducing the risk of injury. Here are some bodyweight exercises that can be included in a core workout:

1. Planks: Planks are a classic exercise that target the core, including the abs, obliques, and lower back. They can be performed in a variety of positions, including standard, side, and decline planks.

2. Sit-ups: Sit-ups are a classic exercise that target the abs and lower back. They can be performed with or without resistance.

3. Russian Twists: Russian twists are an exercise that target the obliques and lower back. To perform a Russian twist, sit on the ground with your knees bent and your feet off the ground. Hold your hands together and twist your torso from side to side.

4. Leg Raises: Leg raises are an exercise that target the lower abs. To perform a leg raise, lie on your back with your hands under your lower back and raise your legs until they are perpendicular to the ground.

5. Bicycle Crunches: Bicycle crunches are an exercise that target the abs and obliques. To perform a bicycle crunch, lie on your back with your hands behind your head and alternate bringing your knee to your elbow.

Lower Body Workouts

Lower body workouts are an effective way to build muscle and increase strength in the legs and glutes. Here are some bodyweight exercises that can be included in a lower body workout:

1. Squats: Squats are a classic exercise that target the legs, glutes, and lower back. There are numerous variations of squats, including bodyweight squats, pistol squats, and jump squats.

2. Lunges: Lunges are an exercise that target the legs, glutes, and hips. They can be performed in a variety of positions, including forward lunges, reverse lunges, and lateral lunges.

3. Leg Press: The leg press is an exercise that targets the legs, glutes, and lower back. To perform a leg press, lie on your back with your hands under your lower back and press your legs into the air.

4. Calf Raises: Calf raises are an exercise that target the calves. To perform a calf raise, stand with your feet hip-width apart and raise and lower your heels.

5. Step-ups: Step-ups are an exercise that target the legs and glutes. To perform a step-up, step onto a sturdy platform or bench with one foot, then step back down with the same foot.

Total Body Workouts

Total body workouts are an effective way to build muscle and increase overall fitness, targeting multiple muscle groups at once. Here are some bodyweight exercises that can be included in a total body workout:

1. Burpees: Burpees are a dynamic exercise that target the chest, triceps, legs, glutes, and core. To perform a burpee, start in a standing position, then lower into a squat, place your hands on the ground, jump your feet back into a plank position, do a push-up, jump your feet back to your hands, and then jump into the air.

2. Jumping Jacks: Jumping jacks are a classic exercise that target the legs, glutes, and core. To perform a jumping jack, start in a standing position, then jump and spread your legs and arms out to the sides, then jump back to the starting position.

3. Mountain Climbers: Mountain climbers are an exercise that target the legs, glutes, and core. To perform a mountain climber, start in a plank position, then alternate bringing your knees to your chest.

4. Squat Jumps: Squat jumps are a dynamic exercise that target the legs, glutes, and core. To perform a squat jump, start in a squat position, then jump into the air, landing back in the squat position.

5. Tuck Jumps: Tuck jumps are a dynamic exercise that target the legs, glutes, and core. To perform a tuck jump, start in a standing position, then jump into the air, bringing your knees to your chest.

Staying Motivated and Overcoming Plateaus

Staying motivated and overcoming plateaus are common challenges when it comes to fitness and bodyweight training. Here are some tips for staying motivated and overcoming plateaus:

1. Set Realistic Goals: Setting realistic goals can help to keep you motivated and on track. Start with small, achievable goals, and gradually increase the difficulty over time.

2. Track Your Progress: Keeping track of your progress, either through a journal or a fitness app, can help to keep you motivated and see the progress you're making.

3. Incorporate Variety: Incorporating variety into your bodyweight workouts can help to prevent boredom and keep you motivated. Try new exercises, change up your routine, and vary the difficulty over time.

4. Get a Workout Buddy: Having a workout buddy can help to keep you accountable and motivated. You can push each other to reach your goals and provide encouragement and support.

5. Celebrate Your Successes: Celebrating your successes, no matter how small, can help to keep you motivated and focused on your goals.

6. Overcoming Plateaus: Plateaus are a natural part of the fitness journey and can be overcome by gradually increasing the difficulty of your exercises, incorporating new exercises, and tracking your progress.

Tracking Progress and Setting New Goals

Tracking progress and setting new goals are important components of bodyweight training and overall fitness. Here are some tips for tracking progress and setting new goals:

1. Track Progress Regularly: Regularly tracking your progress, whether through journaling or using a fitness app, can help you see the progress you're making and stay motivated.

2. Measure Progress Beyond the Scale: While weight loss is an important goal for some, it's important to measure progress beyond just the scale. Consider tracking body measurements, strength improvements, and increases in endurance.

3. Set Realistic Goals: Setting realistic goals is important for maintaining motivation and making progress. Start with achievable goals and gradually increase the difficulty over time.

4. Re-evaluate Goals Regularly: Regularly re-evaluating your goals can help you stay on track and adjust your approach as needed. If you've achieved a goal, set a new one, and continue to push yourself towards improved fitness.

5. Celebrate Your Successes: Celebrating your successes, no matter how small, can help to keep you motivated and focused on your goals.

By tracking progress and setting new goals, you'll be able to stay motivated and make progress on your journey to improved fitness and muscle mass.

Staying Motivated with Support and Community

Staying motivated is an important aspect of bodyweight training and overall fitness, and having support and a sense of community can be incredibly helpful. Here are some tips for staying motivated with support and community:

1. Find a Workout Buddy: Having a workout buddy can help to keep you accountable, provide encouragement and support, and make working out more enjoyable.

2. Join a Fitness Community: Joining a fitness community, whether online or in-person, can help you connect with others who have similar goals and provide a sense of support and camaraderie.

3. Participate in Fitness Challenges: Participating in fitness challenges, whether with friends or in a larger community, can help to keep you motivated and focused on your goals.

4. Hire a Personal Trainer: Hiring a personal trainer can provide you with support, motivation, and personalized advice to help you reach your goals.

5. Share Your Journey: Sharing your journey, whether through social media or with friends and family, can help to keep you accountable and provide a sense of community and support.

By seeking support and community, you'll be able to stay motivated and reach your bodyweight training and fitness goals with greater ease.

Mixing Things Up to Avoid Plateaus

Plateaus are a common challenge in bodyweight training and fitness, but they can be overcome by mixing things up and changing your routine. Here are some tips for avoiding plateaus and continuing to make progress:

1. Increase the Difficulty: Gradually increasing the difficulty of your exercises, whether through reps, sets, or weight, can help you avoid plateaus and continue to make progress.

2. Incorporate New Exercises: Incorporating new exercises into your routine can help to challenge your muscles in new ways and prevent boredom.

3. Vary Your Workouts: Varying your workouts, whether through different exercises, reps, sets, or weights, can help to keep your body challenged and prevent plateaus.

4. Change Your Workout Environment: Changing your workout environment, whether through outdoor workouts or new locations, can help to keep you motivated and prevent boredom.

5. Set New Goals: Setting new goals, whether for strength, endurance, or weight loss, can help to keep you motivated and focused on your journey.

By mixing things up and changing your routine, you'll be able to avoid plateaus and continue to make progress on your journey to improved fitness and muscle mass.

Nutrition for Building Muscle at 50

Proper nutrition is an important aspect of bodyweight training and building muscle, especially as we age. Here are some tips for optimizing your nutrition for building muscle at 50:

1. Eat Enough Protein: Protein is essential for building muscle, so make sure to include adequate amounts of protein in your diet. Good sources of protein include lean meats, poultry, fish, eggs, and dairy products.

2. Consume Adequate Carbohydrates: Carbohydrates provide energy for workouts and support muscle recovery, so make sure to include adequate amounts of carbohydrates in your diet. Good sources of carbohydrates include fruits, vegetables, whole grains, and legumes.

3. Include Healthy Fats: Healthy fats, such as those found in nuts, seeds, and avocados, are important for overall health and can help to support muscle building.

4. Stay Hydrated: Staying hydrated is important for overall health and can help to support muscle recovery and performance. Aim to drink at least 8 glasses of water a day.

5. Limit Processed Foods and Added Sugars: Processed foods and added sugars can be high in empty calories and can interfere with muscle building efforts. Limit your intake of these foods and opt for whole, nutrient-dense foods instead.

By following these nutrition tips, you'll be able to optimize your nutrition for building muscle at 50 and support your bodyweight training efforts.

The Importance of Protein for Muscle Growth

Protein is an essential nutrient for muscle growth and recovery, especially for those engaging in bodyweight training. Here's why protein is so important:

1. Building and Repairing Tissues: Protein is essential for building and repairing tissues, including muscle tissue. When you engage in bodyweight training, you create small tears in your muscle fibers, and protein is needed to repair and build these fibers back up.

2. Stimulating Muscle Protein Synthesis: Protein stimulates muscle protein synthesis, which is the process by which your body builds new muscle tissue. Consuming enough protein is essential for maximizing muscle growth and recovery.

3. Supporting Hormonal Responses: Protein is also important for supporting hormonal responses in the body that are essential for muscle growth. For example, consuming protein can help to increase levels of the hormone testosterone, which is important for muscle growth.

4. Maintaining Muscle Mass: As we age, we naturally lose muscle mass, and consuming adequate amounts of protein can help to slow this process and maintain muscle mass.

By consuming enough protein, you'll be able to support muscle growth and recovery, and maximize the benefits of your bodyweight training efforts. Aim to consume at least

0.8 grams of protein per kilogram of body weight per day to support muscle growth and recovery.

Eating for Energy and Endurance

Eating a balanced and nutritious diet can provide the energy and endurance needed for bodyweight training and other physical activities. Here are some tips for eating for energy and endurance:

1. Consume Adequate Carbohydrates: Carbohydrates are the primary source of energy for the body, and consuming adequate amounts of carbohydrates can help to provide the energy needed for physical activity. Good sources of carbohydrates include fruits, vegetables, whole grains, and legumes.

2. Include Healthy Fats: Healthy fats, such as those found in nuts, seeds, and avocados, can provide sustained energy and support overall health.

3. Stay Hydrated: Staying hydrated is important for overall health and can help to support endurance and performance. Aim to drink at least 8 glasses of water a day.

4. Eat Enough Protein: Protein is essential for building and repairing muscle tissue, and consuming adequate amounts of protein can help to support muscle growth and recovery.

5. Limit Processed Foods and Added Sugars: Processed foods and added sugars can be high in empty calories and can interfere with energy levels and endurance. Limit your intake of these foods and opt for whole, nutrient-dense foods instead.

By following these nutrition tips, you'll be able to eat for energy and endurance, and support your bodyweight training and physical activities.

Hydration and Supplements for Optimal Performance

Proper hydration and the use of supplements can play a role in supporting optimal performance during bodyweight training and other physical activities. Here are some tips for hydration and supplement use:

1. Stay Hydrated: Staying hydrated is essential for overall health and performance, and can help to support endurance and recovery. Aim to drink at least 8 glasses of water a day, and more before, during, and after physical activity.

2. Consider Sports Drinks: Sports drinks can be helpful for replenishing electrolytes lost through sweat and supporting hydration during prolonged physical activity.

3. Use Supplements Wisely: Supplements can be helpful for supporting muscle growth and recovery, but it's important to use them wisely. Consult with a healthcare professional before starting any new supplement regimen, and opt for high-quality supplements with minimal added ingredients.

4. Focus on Whole Foods: While supplements can be helpful, it's important to focus on a balanced diet of whole, nutrient-dense foods as the foundation of your nutrition.

By staying hydrated and using supplements wisely, you'll be able to support optimal performance during bodyweight training and other physical activities.

Conclusion

Bodyweight training can be a highly effective way to build muscle and improve fitness, especially for men over 50. By following the principles of progressive resistance training, incorporating variety into your workouts, staying motivated and overcoming plateaus, and optimizing your nutrition, you'll be able to reach your goals and achieve improved fitness and muscle mass.

In addition, proper hydration and the wise use of supplements can play a role in supporting optimal performance during bodyweight training and other physical activities. By following these tips and recommendations, you'll be well on your way to a successful and fulfilling fitness journey.

Celebrating Your Achievements

Celebrating your achievements is an important aspect of bodyweight training and overall fitness. Here are some tips for celebrating your achievements:

1. Set and Achieve Realistic Goals: Setting realistic goals and achieving them can provide a sense of accomplishment and satisfaction.

2. Track Your Progress: Keeping track of your progress, whether through journaling or a fitness app, can help you see the progress you're making and provide a sense of accomplishment.

3. Celebrate Small Wins: Celebrating small wins, such as hitting a new personal best, can help to keep you motivated and focused on your goals.

4. Recognize Your Efforts: Recognizing your efforts and the hard work you've put into your fitness journey can help to provide a sense of satisfaction and accomplishment.

5. Treat Yourself: Treating yourself to something you enjoy, such as a massage or a new workout outfit, can help to celebrate your achievements and provide a sense of reward.

By celebrating your achievements, you'll be able to stay motivated and focused on your fitness journey, and enjoy the satisfaction of reaching your goals.

Staying Committed to Your Fitness Journey

Staying committed to your fitness journey can be challenging, but it's an important aspect of achieving your goals. Here are some tips for staying committed to your fitness journey:

1. Set Realistic Goals: Setting realistic goals can help to keep you motivated and on track. Start with small, achievable goals, and gradually increase the difficulty over time.

2. Make a Plan: Having a plan, including a schedule for workouts and meal planning, can help to keep you accountable and focused on your goals.

3. Find a Workout Buddy: Having a workout buddy can provide accountability, encouragement, and support, and make working out more enjoyable.

4. Incorporate Variety: Incorporating variety into your workouts, whether through new exercises, changing your routine, or varying the difficulty, can help to keep you motivated and prevent boredom.

5. Celebrate Your Successes: Celebrating your successes, no matter how small, can help to keep you motivated and focused on your goals.

By staying committed to your fitness journey, you'll be able to reach your goals and enjoy the benefits of improved fitness and muscle mass.

Sample Workout Plans

Here are three sample workout plans for men over 50 looking to build muscle with bodyweight exercises:

Plan 1: Upper Body Focus

- Warm-up: 5-10 minutes of light cardio, such as jogging or jumping jacks
- Push-ups: 3 sets of 12-15 reps
- Dips: 3 sets of 12-15 reps
- Diamond push-ups: 3 sets of 12-15 reps
- Plank: 3 sets, holding for 30-60 seconds
- Cool-down: 5-10 minutes of stretching

Plan 2: Core Focus

- Warm-up: 5-10 minutes of light cardio, such as jogging or jumping jacks
- Crunches: 3 sets of 12-15 reps
- Bicycle crunches: 3 sets of 12-15 reps
- Leg raises: 3 sets of 12-15 reps
- Russian twists: 3 sets of 12-15 reps
- Cool-down: 5-10 minutes of stretching

Plan 3: Total Body Focus

- Warm-up: 5-10 minutes of light cardio, such as jogging or jumping jacks

- Push-ups: 3 sets of 12-15 reps

- Squats: 3 sets of 12-15 reps

- Lunges: 3 sets of 12-15 reps

- Plank: 3 sets, holding for 30-60 seconds

- Cool-down: 5-10 minutes of stretching

These sample workout plans are a starting point and can be adjusted to suit your individual needs and goals. By incorporating a variety of exercises and regularly changing up your routine, you'll be able to challenge your muscles in new ways and continue to make progress on your fitness journey.

Glossary of Terms.

1. Bodyweight Training: A form of resistance training that uses the weight of one's own body as resistance, rather than external weights.

2. Progressive Resistance Training: A method of strength training that involves gradually increasing the weight or resistance used in exercises over time to continually challenge the muscles and promote growth.

3. Plateau: A period of time during which progress in strength or fitness appears to stall or slow.

4. Muscle Protein Synthesis: The process by which the body builds new muscle tissue.

5. Electrolytes: Minerals, such as sodium, potassium, and magnesium, that are important for maintaining fluid balance and supporting overall health and performance.

6. Testosterone: A hormone that is important for muscle growth and overall health.

7. Supplements: Products, such as vitamins, minerals, or amino acids, that are taken in addition to a normal diet to support overall health and performance.

8. Plateau Busting: Strategies for overcoming a period of time during which progress appears to stall or slow.

By understanding these terms, you'll be better equipped to navigate your bodyweight training journey and achieve your goals.